ROTH.S

Strength and Flexibility: Resistance Band Workouts for Seniors

First edition

This book was professionally typeset on Reedsy.
Find out more at reedsy.com

Contents

1

Introduction

Welcome to a Stronger, More Flexible You

Imagine waking up each morning feeling energized, strong, and ready to tackle the day. Picture yourself moving with ease, free from the stiffness and aches that often accompany aging. This is not just a dream—it's an achievable reality. Welcome to "Strength and Flexibility: Resistance Band Workouts for Seniors."

Why This Book?

As we age, maintaining our physical health becomes increasingly important. Yet, many seniors struggle to find safe and effective ways to stay active. This book was born out of a desire to address this need. Written with seniors in mind, it provides simple, step-by-step instructions for using resistance bands to improve strength and flexibility. These lightweight, portable tools can transform your fitness routine, offering a gentle yet powerful way to build muscle and enhance mobility.

What You'll Learn

This book is designed to be your go-to guide for resistance band workouts. Whether you're a complete beginner or have some experience with exercise, you'll find valuable insights and routines that suit your needs. Here's a glimpse of what we'll cover:

- **Choosing the Right Bands**: Learn how to select the best resistance bands for your fitness level and goals.
- **Warm-Up**: Discover effective warm-up routines to prepare your body for exercise.
- **Upper Body Workouts**: Strengthen your arms, shoulders, and chest with targeted exercises.
- **Lower Body Workouts**: Build strength in your legs and hips, improving balance and mobility.
- **Core Strengthening**: Enhance your core stability with exercises that support overall strength.
- **Flexibility and Stretching**: Increase your range of motion and reduce stiffness with gentle stretches.
- **Cool Down and Recovery**: Learn how to properly cool down and aid recovery after workouts.
- **Maintaining Motivation**: Find tips and strategies to stay motivated and consistent with your exercise routine.

How This Book Will Benefit You

By following the routines and advice in this book, you'll gain:

- **Improved Strength**: Build muscle to support everyday activities and reduce the risk of falls.
- **Enhanced Flexibility**: Increase your range of motion, making

movements more fluid and comfortable.

- **Better Balance**: Strengthen key muscle groups that contribute to stability and prevent falls.
- **Greater Independence**: Stay active and self-reliant, enjoying a higher quality of life.
- **Boosted Confidence**: Feel more confident in your physical abilities and overall health.

The Benefits of Resistance Band Workouts

Resistance bands offer numerous benefits for seniors, including:

- **Safety:** Low-impact exercises reduce the risk of injury.
- **Convenience:** You can work out at home, at your own pace.
- **Versatility:** Bands can be used for a wide range of exercises targeting different muscle groups.
- **Cost-Effectiveness:** Resistance bands are affordable and durable.

Your Path to a Healthier Life

Embarking on this fitness journey will not only improve your physical health but also boost your confidence and overall well-being. The workouts in this book are designed to be simple, effective, and adaptable to your individual needs. Remember, it's never too late to start, and every small step you take brings you closer to a healthier, more active lifestyle.

2

Choosing the Right Bands

The Importance of the Right Equipment

Starting your fitness journey with the right tools is crucial for success and safety. In this chapter, we will explore how to choose the right resistance bands for your needs, where you can buy them and what the cost of the bands are and how to use them safely.

Understanding Your Options

When selecting resistance bands for seniors, it's important to consider factors such as ease of use, safety, and appropriate resistance levels. Here are some recommendations:

1. **Light to Medium Resistance**: Seniors should opt for bands that offer light to medium resistance. These bands provide enough tension for effective exercise without causing strain or injury.
2. **Flat Bands or Loop Bands**: Flat bands (also known as Therabands) and loop bands are generally easier to handle and less intimidating

4

for seniors compared to tube bands with handles.

3. **Comfortable Material**: Look for bands made from high-quality, comfortable material that is gentle on the skin. Latex-free options are available for those with allergies.
4. **Colour-Coded Resistance Levels**: Many resistance bands come in color-coded sets that indicate different resistance levels. This makes it easier to select the appropriate band and track progress.
5. **Non-Slip Grip**: Bands with a non-slip grip can prevent slipping during exercises, enhancing safety.
6. **Safety Features**: Ensure the bands have reinforced ends or attachments to prevent snapping or breaking during use.
7. **Portability**: Lightweight and portable bands are beneficial as they can be easily used at home or taken to fitness classes.

Recommended Brands and Types:

1. **TheraBand Professional Latex Resistance Bands**: These are popular among physical therapists and come in a range of resistance levels, making them suitable for seniors.
2. **Fit Simplify Resistance Loop Exercise Bands**: These loop bands are color-coded for different resistance levels and come with instructional materials.
3. **SPRI Xertube Resistance Bands with Handles**: These bands have a more secure grip with handles, suitable for those who prefer more control during exercises.
4. **Bodylastics Resistance Bands Set**: Known for their durability and safety features, these bands come with a variety of attachments and handles.

It's always a good idea for seniors to consult with a healthcare provider or physical therapist before starting any new exercise program to ensure that the chosen resistance bands and exercises are appropriate for their individual fitness levels and health conditions.

Where to Buy Resistance Bands

You can purchase resistance bands from a variety of places, both online and in-store:

Online Retailers

- **Amazon:** A wide selection of resistance bands in various types and resistance levels. Prices range from $10 to $30 for sets.
- **Walmart:** Offers affordable options, often with in-store pickup or delivery. Sets typically range from $10 to $25.
- **Specialty Fitness Stores:** Websites like Rogue Fitness or Perform Better offer high-quality bands, usually priced from $15 to $40.

Physical Stores

- **Sporting Goods Stores:** Stores like Dick's Sporting Goods or Academy Sports + Outdoors have a variety of resistance bands. Prices here can range from $10 to $30.
- **Department Stores:** Places like Target or Walmart also carry resistance bands in their fitness sections, often at very competitive prices.

Tips for Saving Money

Here are some tips to help you save money when buying resistance bands:

- **Buy Sets:** Purchasing a set of bands that includes multiple resistance levels is often cheaper than buying them individually.
- **Look for Sales:** Keep an eye out for sales, especially around holidays or end-of-season clearances.
- **Read Reviews:** Check customer reviews to ensure you're getting a quality product. Sometimes cheaper bands can wear out quickly.
- **Consider Bundles:** Some bands come with additional equipment like handles, door anchors, or workout guides, which can add value.

Basic Equipment Needed

To enhance your resistance band workouts and ensure you exercise safely and effectively, a few additional pieces of equipment can be very helpful. Here's a detailed look at the basic equipment you'll need and why each item is important.

A Sturdy Chair

A sturdy chair is essential for performing seated exercises or providing support during standing exercises. It helps maintain balance and stability, particularly for seniors who may need extra support. Ensure the chair is stable and without wheels to prevent slipping. Using a chair can make exercises more accessible and reduce the risk of falls, allowing you to focus on performing each movement correctly and safely.

Exercise Mat

An exercise mat provides cushioning and support for floor exercises. It prevents slipping and adds comfort, especially when performing exercises on hard surfaces. A good mat will also protect your joints by providing a softer surface to work on. This is particularly important for exercises that require kneeling or lying down, helping to prevent discomfort and injury.

Comfortable Clothing and Footwear

Wearing comfortable, non-restrictive clothing is crucial for allowing free movement during exercises. Choose breathable fabrics that wick away moisture to keep you cool and comfortable. Supportive footwear is equally important as it helps maintain balance and prevent slips, especially during standing exercises. Proper shoes can provide the necessary grip and support to perform exercises more effectively and safely.

Door Anchor

A door anchor is a small but incredibly useful accessory for resistance band workouts. It allows you to secure your band to a door, creating a stable anchor point for various exercises. This expands the range of exercises you can perform, enabling you to work different muscle groups more effectively. Ensure the door you use is sturdy and that the anchor is securely attached to avoid accidents.

Foam Roller

A foam roller is a great tool for muscle recovery and flexibility. Using a foam roller before and after workouts can help relieve muscle tension, improve blood flow, and enhance flexibility. It's particularly useful for seniors as it aids in reducing stiffness and promoting better mobility. Incorporating foam rolling into your routine can help prevent injuries and improve overall exercise performance.

Water Bottle

Staying hydrated is crucial during any form of exercise. Keeping a water bottle nearby ensures you can easily stay hydrated throughout your workout. Proper hydration helps maintain energy levels and supports muscle function, which is essential for effective exercise. Make it a habit to take small sips of water regularly to stay well-hydrated.

Resistance Band Handles

Handles can be attached to tube bands to make them easier to grip, especially during upper body exercises. They provide a more comfortable and secure hold, allowing you to focus on the movement without worrying about the band slipping. Handles can also help distribute the resistance more evenly across your hands, making exercises more effective.

Having the right equipment can significantly enhance your resistance band workouts, making them safer and more effective. Each piece of equipment serves a specific purpose, from providing support and comfort to expanding the range of exercises you can perform. By investing in these basic items, you'll be well-prepared to embark on your fitness journey with confidence. In the next chapter, we'll cover the importance of warming up and provide simple warm-up routines to prepare your body for exercise.

3

Warm-Up

The Importance and Benefits of a Warm-Up Routine

Starting your workout with a proper warm-up is essential for preparing your body for the physical activity ahead. A good warm-up gradually increases your heart rate and blood flow to your muscles, which helps to prevent injuries and improve your overall performance. For seniors, warming up is particularly important as it helps to loosen joints, improve flexibility, and reduce muscle stiffness. By spending a few minutes warming up, you can ensure a safer and more effective workout.

Warm-Up Exercises: Step by Step

To get the most out of your warm-up, follow these step-by-step exercises designed to gently prepare your entire body for exercise.

Marching in Place

1. Stand with your feet hip-width apart.
2. Begin to march in place, lifting your knees as high as comfortable.
3. Swing your arms naturally with each step.
4. Continue for 1-2 minutes, gradually increasing the speed as you feel more comfortable.

Arm Circles

1. Stand with your feet shoulder-width apart and extend your arms out to the sides at shoulder height.
2. Begin to make small circles with your arms, gradually increasing the size of the circles.
3. After about 30 seconds, reverse the direction of the circles.
4. Continue for another 30 seconds.

Leg Swings

1. Stand beside a sturdy chair or wall for support.
2. Gently swing one leg forward and backward, keeping your movements smooth and controlled.
3. Perform 10-15 swings on each leg.
4. Switch to the other leg and repeat.

Shoulder Shrugs

1. Stand with your feet shoulder-width apart.
2. Lift your shoulders towards your ears, hold for a few seconds, and then relax them back down.
3. Repeat this movement 10-15 times.

Ankle Circles

1. Sit in a sturdy chair or stand while holding onto something for balance.
2. Lift one foot off the ground and gently rotate your ankle in a circular motion.
3. Perform 10-15 circles in one direction, then reverse the direction.
4. Switch to the other ankle and repeat.

Gentle Side Bends

1. Stand with your feet shoulder-width apart and place your hands on your hips.
2. Slowly bend to one side, reaching your hand down towards your knee while keeping your upper body straight.
3. Return to the center and bend to the other side.
4. Repeat 10 times on each side.

Whole Body Warm-Up

For a comprehensive warm-up that prepares your entire body, combine the exercises listed above into a single routine. This will ensure all major muscle groups are engaged and ready for your workout. Here's a suggested sequence:

1. **Marching in Place:** 2 minutes
2. **Arm Circles:** 1 minute (30 seconds each direction)
3. **Leg Swings:** 1 minute (30 seconds per leg)
4. **Shoulder Shrugs:** 1 minute
5. **Ankle Circles:** 1 minute (30 seconds per ankle)
6. **Gentle Side Bends:** 2 minutes (1 minute per side)

A proper warm-up routine is the foundation of a safe and effective workout. By incorporating these simple exercises, you can prepare your body for the physical activity ahead, reducing the risk of injury and enhancing your performance. Remember to take your time and focus on smooth, controlled movements. In the next chapter, we will dive into upper body workouts using resistance bands, providing you with effective exercises to strengthen your arms, shoulders, and chest.

4

Upper Body Workout

Strengthening Your Upper Body

B uilding strength in your upper body is essential for daily activities and overall fitness. This chapter will guide you through a series of exercises targeting your shoulders, arms, and chest, providing detailed instructions to ensure you perform each exercise correctly and safely.

Shoulder Exercises

Front Shoulder Raise

1. **Starting Position:** Stand with your feet shoulder-width apart, holding a resistance band with both hands in front of you, palms facing down.
2. **Execution:** Slowly lift your arms straight in front of you until they are parallel to the floor, keeping a slight bend in your elbows.
3. **Hold:** Pause for a second at the top.

4. **Return:** Lower your arms back to the starting position in a controlled manner.
5. **Repetitions:** Perform 10-15 repetitions.

Lateral Shoulder Raise

1. **Starting Position:** Stand with your feet shoulder-width apart, holding the resistance band with both hands at your sides, palms facing inward.
2. **Execution:** Lift your arms out to the sides until they are parallel to the floor, maintaining a slight bend in your elbows.
3. **Hold:** Pause for a second at the top.
4. **Return:** Slowly lower your arms back to the starting position.
5. **Repetitions:** Perform 10-15 repetitions.

Shoulder Press

1. **Starting Position:** Stand with your feet shoulder-width apart, holding the resistance band handles at shoulder height with your palms facing forward.
2. **Execution:** Push your hands upward until your arms are fully extended above your head.
3. **Hold:** Pause for a second at the top.
4. **Return:** Lower your hands back to the starting position in a controlled manner.
5. **Repetitions:** Perform 10-15 repetitions.

Overhead band pull-apart

1. **Starting Position:** Hold the band straight above your head.
2. **Execution:** Pull the band apart as you lower your arms to shoulder height, pressing your hands out to the sides.
3. **Hold:** Hold this position for a few seconds.
4. **Return:** Slowly return to the starting position, aiming to keep your shoulder blades down, away from your ears.
5. **Repetitions:** Perform 10-15 repetitions. For added intensity, use a band with higher resistance or perform the exercise more slowly.

This exercise targets your shoulders, back, and triceps. It improves stability, mobility, and posture.

Strengthening your shoulders with these resistance band exercises will improve your upper body mobility and functionality. By following these step-by-step instructions, you can safely and effectively target your shoulder muscles. In the next section, we will focus on arm exercises to further enhance your upper body strength.

Arm Exercises

Strengthening your arms is crucial for many daily activities, from lifting groceries to pushing a lawnmower. This section will guide you through four effective resistance band exercises for your arms: Bicep Curls, Tricep Extensions, Hammer Curls, and Overhead Tricep Extensions.

Bicep Curls

Bicep curls target the muscles at the front of your upper arm, helping you build strength for tasks that involve lifting or carrying objects.

1. **Starting Position:** Stand with your feet shoulder-width apart, stepping on the middle of the resistance band. Hold the handles or ends of the band with your palms facing forward, arms fully extended down by your sides.
2. **Execution:** Slowly curl your hands toward your shoulders, bending at the elbows and keeping your upper arms stationary. Focus on squeezing your biceps at the top of the movement.
3. **Hold:** Pause for a second at the top of the curl.
4. **Return:** Lower your hands back to the starting position in a controlled manner, resisting the band's pull.
5. **Repetitions:** Perform 10-15 repetitions. For added challenge, increase the resistance of the band or perform the exercise more slowly.

Tricep Extensions

Tricep extensions target the muscles at the back of your upper arm, essential for pushing movements and overall arm strength.

1. **Starting Position:** Stand with one foot slightly in front of the other, holding the resistance band in both hands behind your head, elbows bent. Ensure the band is secure and taut.
2. **Execution:** Extend your arms upward, straightening your elbows and keeping your upper arms close to your head.
3. **Hold:** Pause for a second at the top of the extension.
4. **Return:** Lower your hands back to the starting position in a controlled manner, ensuring you feel the tension in your triceps.
5. **Repetitions:** Perform 10-15 repetitions. If you find it too easy, try using a band with higher resistance or perform the movement more slowly.

Hammer Curls

Hammer curls focus on the brachialis muscle, which lies underneath the biceps and helps to increase the overall size and strength of the upper arm.

1. **Starting Position:** Stand with your feet shoulder-width apart, stepping on the middle of the resistance band. Hold the handles or ends of the band with your palms facing inward, arms fully extended down by your sides.
2. **Execution:** Curl your hands toward your shoulders, maintaining your palms facing each other throughout the movement.
3. **Hold:** Pause for a second at the top of the curl.
4. Return: Lower your hands back to the starting position in a controlled manner, resisting the band's pull.
5. Repetitions: Perform 10-15 repetitions.

Overhead Tricep Extensions

This exercise targets the triceps and involves a different movement pattern, adding variety to your arm workout.

1. **Starting Position:** Stand with your feet shoulder-width apart, stepping on the middle of the resistance band. Hold the handles or ends of the band with your hands behind your head, elbows bent.
2. **Execution:** Extend your arms upward, fully straightening your elbows. Keep your upper arms close to your head.
3. **Hold:** Pause for a second at the top of the extension.
4. **Return:** Lower your hands back to the starting position in a controlled manner.
5. **Repetitions:** Perform 10-15 repetitions.

Incorporating these arm exercises into your routine will help you build strength and improve the functionality of your upper body. By following these detailed instructions, you can ensure you are performing the exercises safely and effectively. In the next section, we will explore chest exercises to further enhance your upper body workout.

Chest Exercises

Building a strong chest is essential for many daily activities, from pushing open doors to lifting objects. This section will guide you through four effective resistance band exercises for your chest: Chest Press, Chest Fly, Push-Ups with Resistance Bands, and Standing Chest Squeeze.

Chest Press

The chest press targets the pectoral muscles, helping to build strength and endurance in your upper body.

1. **Starting Position:** Secure the resistance band behind you at chest level (using a door anchor or wrapping it around a sturdy object). Stand with your feet shoulder-width apart, holding the handles or ends of the band with your elbows bent and hands at chest level.
2. **Execution:** Push your hands forward until your arms are fully extended, keeping them at chest height. Your palms should face down as you press forward.
3. **Hold:** Pause for a second at the top of the movement, feeling the contraction in your chest muscles.
4. **Return:** Slowly bring your hands back to the starting position in

a controlled manner, resisting the band's pull.

5. **Repetitions:** Perform 10-15 repetitions. If you need more of a challenge, use a band with higher resistance or increase the number of repetitions.

Chest Fly

The chest fly is an excellent exercise for targeting the inner part of your chest muscles, providing a great stretch and strengthening the chest.

1. **Starting Position:** Secure the resistance band behind you at chest level. Stand with your feet shoulder-width apart, holding the handles or ends of the band with your arms extended out to the sides, elbows slightly bent, and palms facing forward.
2. **Execution:** Bring your hands together in front of your chest in a wide, hugging motion, keeping a slight bend in your elbows throughout the movement.
3. **Hold:** Pause for a second when your hands meet in front of your chest, squeezing your chest muscles.
4. **Return:** Slowly move your arms back to the starting position, maintaining control and resisting the band's pull.
5. **Repetitions:** Perform 10-15 repetitions. For added intensity, use a band with higher resistance or perform the exercise more slowly.

Push-Ups with Resistance Bands

Adding resistance bands to push-ups increases the intensity and targets your chest muscles more effectively.

1. **Starting Position:** Loop the resistance band around your back and hold the ends in your hands. Get into a push-up position with

your hands slightly wider than shoulder-width apart and your feet
together.

2. **Execution:** Lower your body until your chest nearly touches the
floor, keeping your elbows at about a 45-degree angle to your body.

3. **Hold:** Pause briefly at the bottom.

4. **Return:** Push back up to the starting position, extending your
arms fully and feeling the resistance from the band.

5. **Repetitions:** Perform 8-12 repetitions. Adjust the resistance of
the band or your hand placement to modify the difficulty.

Standing Chest Squeeze

This exercise targets your chest muscles through an isometric hold,
helping to build endurance and strength.

1. **Starting Position:** Stand with your feet shoulder-width apart,
holding the resistance band in front of you with both hands, arms
extended straight.

2. **Execution:** Pull the band apart slightly to create tension, then
bring your hands together in front of your chest, squeezing your
chest muscles as if you're trying to crush something between your
hands.

3. **Hold:** Maintain the squeeze for 5-10 seconds, focusing on contracting your chest muscles.

4. **Return:** Release the tension slightly without fully relaxing your
muscles.

5. **Repetitions:** Perform 8-10 repetitions, holding each squeeze for
a few seconds.

Incorporating these chest exercises into your workout routine will help you build strength and improve the functionality of your upper body. By following these detailed instructions, you can ensure you are performing the exercises safely and effectively. In the next chapter, we will explore core strengthening exercises to enhance your overall stability and balance.

5

Lower Body Workout

Building Strength in Your Lower Body

Strengthening your lower body is essential for maintaining mobility and performing daily activities with ease. This chapter will guide you through a series of exercises targeting your legs, hips, and glute, providing detailed instructions and step-by-step guidance to ensure you perform each exercise correctly and safely.

Exercises for Legs

Strengthening your legs is crucial for maintaining mobility and independence in daily activities. Here are four effective resistance band exercises designed for seniors to improve leg strength, balance, and stability.

Squats with Resistance Bands

Squats target the quadriceps, hamstrings, and glute, improving overall lower body strength.

1. **Starting Position:** Stand with your feet shoulder-width apart, stepping on the middle of the resistance band. Hold the handles or ends of the band at shoulder height with your elbows bent.
2. **Execution:** Lower your body as if you are sitting back into a chair, keeping your back straight and your knees over your toes.
3. **Hold:** Pause for a second at the bottom of the squat.
4. **Return:** Push through your heels to return to the starting position, straightening your legs.
5. **Repetitions:** Perform 10-15 repetitions. Use a band with higher resistance or perform the exercise more slowly for added challenge.

Leg Press with Resistance Bands

The leg press targets your quadriceps, hamstrings, and glutes, helping to build strength and endurance in your lower body.

1. **Starting Position:** Sit on the floor with your legs extended in front of you, looping the resistance band around the soles of your feet. Hold the handles or ends of the band with your hands at your sides.
2. **Execution:** Push your feet away from your body, straightening your legs against the resistance of the band.
3. **Hold:** Pause for a second at the top of the movement, fully extending your legs.
4. **Return:** Slowly bend your knees to return to the starting position, keeping the band taut.

5. **Repetitions:** Perform 10-15 repetitions. Adjust the resistance of the band to modify the difficulty.

Seated Leg Extensions

Leg extensions specifically target the quadriceps, enhancing strength and stability in the knee joint.

1. **Starting Position:** Sit on a sturdy chair with your back straight and feet flat on the floor. Loop the resistance band around one foot and hold the ends of the band in your hands.
2. **Execution:** Extend your leg straight out in front of you, pulling against the resistance of the band.
3. **Hold:** Pause for a second when your leg is fully extended.
4. **Return:** Slowly lower your leg back to the starting position.
5. **Repetitions:** Perform 10-15 repetitions on each leg. Use a band with higher resistance for added challenge.

Standing Calf Raises with Resistance Bands

Calf raises strengthen the muscles in the lower leg, improving balance and stability.

1. **Starting Position:** Stand with your feet shoulder-width apart, stepping on the middle of the resistance band. Hold the handles or ends of the band at your sides.
2. **Execution:** Raise your heels off the ground, standing on your toes and stretching the band.
3. **Hold:** Pause for a second at the top of the movement.
4. **Return:** Slowly lower your heels back to the starting position.
5. **Repetitions:** Perform 10-15 repetitions. For added difficulty,

increase the resistance of the band or perform the exercise more slowly.

Incorporating these leg exercises into your routine will help you build strength and improve your lower body mobility. By following these detailed, step-by-step instructions, you can ensure you are performing the exercises safely and effectively. In the next section, we will focus on exercises for the hips to further enhance your lower body strength and stability.

Glute Exercises

Strengthening your glute is essential for improving your lower body strength, stability, and overall mobility. Here are four effective resistance band exercises designed for seniors to target the glute, ensuring safe and productive workouts.

Glute Bridges with Resistance Bands

Glute bridges are excellent for targeting the glute and improving hip mobility and lower back strength.

1. **Starting Position:** Lie on your back with your knees bent and feet flat on the floor, shoulder-width apart. Place a loop band just above your knees.
2. **Execution:** Lift your hips towards the ceiling, squeezing your glutes and keeping your shoulders on the floor.
3. **Hold:** Pause for a second at the top of the movement.
4. **Return:** Lower your hips back to the starting position in a controlled manner.
5. **Repetitions:** Perform 10-15 repetitions. For added challenge,

increase the resistance of the band or hold the position longer at the top.

Standing Glute Kickbacks

Glute kickbacks effectively target the glute and hamstrings, enhancing strength and stability.

1. **Starting Position:** Stand with your feet shoulder-width apart, placing a loop band around your ankles. Hold onto a sturdy chair or wall for balance.
2. **Execution:** Extend one leg straight back, keeping your knee straight and foot flexed, feeling the tension in your glute.
3. **Hold:** Pause for a second at the top of the movement.
4. **Return:** Slowly bring your leg back to the starting position.
5. **Repetitions:** Perform 10-15 repetitions on each leg. Use a band with higher resistance for added difficulty.

Side-Lying Leg Lifts

Side-lying leg lifts target the glute and outer thighs, helping to improve hip stability and strength.

1. **Starting Position:** Lie on your side with your legs stacked and a loop band around your ankles. Support your head with one hand.
2. **Execution:** Lift your top leg as high as possible, keeping it straight and maintaining tension in the band.
3. **Hold:** Pause for a second at the top of the movement.
4. **Return:** Slowly lower your leg back to the starting position.
5. **Repetitions:** Perform 10-15 repetitions on each leg. For added challenge, increase the resistance of the band or hold the position

longer at the top.

Clam shells

Clam shells are great for targeting the glute and hip abductors, improving hip strength and stability.

1. **Starting Position:** Lie on your side with your legs bent at a 90-degree angle and a loop band placed just above your knees. Keep your feet together.
2. **Execution:** Lift your top knee as high as you can while keeping your feet together, opening your legs like a clam shell.
3. **Hold:** Pause for a second at the top of the movement.
4. **Return:** Slowly lower your knee back to the starting position.
5. **Repetitions:** Perform 10-15 repetitions on each side. Use a band with higher resistance for added difficulty.

Hip Exercises for Seniors

Strengthening your hips is vital for maintaining balance, stability, and mobility. Here are four effective resistance band exercises designed for seniors to target the hip muscles, ensuring safe and productive workouts.

Hip Abductions with Resistance Bands

Hip abductions strengthen the muscles on the outer sides of your hips, improving stability and balance.

1. **Starting Position:** Stand with your feet hip-width apart, placing a loop band just above your knees. Hold onto a sturdy chair or

wall for balance.

2. **Execution:** Lift one leg out to the side, keeping it straight and maintaining tension in the band.
3. **Hold:** Pause for a second at the top of the movement.
4. **Return:** Slowly lower your leg back to the starting position.
5. **Repetitions:** Perform 10-15 repetitions on each leg. Use a band with higher resistance for added difficulty.

Hip Extensions with Resistance Bands

Hip extensions target the glute and hamstrings, improving lower body strength and posture.

1. **Starting Position:** Stand with your feet shoulder-width apart, stepping on the middle of the resistance band. Hold the handles or ends of the band at your hips.
2. **Execution:** Extend one leg straight back, keeping your knee straight and your foot flexed.
3. **Hold:** Pause for a second at the top of the movement.
4. **Return:** Slowly lower your leg back to the starting position.
5. **Repetitions:** Perform 10-15 repetitions on each leg.

Seated Hip Marches

Seated hip marches help to strengthen the hip flexors and improve hip mobility.

1. **Starting Position:** Sit on a sturdy chair with your back straight and feet flat on the floor. Place a loop band around your thighs, just above your knees.
2. **Execution:** Lift one knee toward your chest, maintaining tension

in the band.
3. **Hold:** Pause for a second at the top of the movement.
4. **Return:** Slowly lower your leg back to the starting position.
5. **Repetitions:** Perform 10-15 repetitions on each leg.

Standing Hip Flexion

Standing hip flexion targets the hip flexors and helps improve balance and strength.

1. **Starting Position:** Stand with your feet hip-width apart, placing a loop band around your ankles. Hold onto a sturdy chair or wall for balance.
2. **Execution:** Lift one knee toward your chest, keeping your leg bent at a 90-degree angle.
3. **Hold:** Pause for a second at the top of the movement.
4. **Return:** Slowly lower your leg back to the starting position.

Repetitions: Perform 10-15 repetitions on each leg. Use a band with higher resistance for added challenge.

6

Core Strengthening

The Importance of a Strong Core

A strong core is essential for overall stability and balance, which are crucial for performing daily activities safely and effectively. Core strengthening exercises help to stabilize your spine, improve posture, and reduce the risk of falls and injuries. This chapter will guide you through a series of exercises designed to strengthen your core, providing detailed instructions and step-by-step guidance to ensure you perform each exercise correctly and safely.

Core Strengthening Exercises

Seated Band Rotations

Seated band rotations target the oblique muscles, which are important for rotational movements and overall core stability.

1. **Starting Position:** Sit on a sturdy chair with your back straight

and feet flat on the floor. Hold the resistance band with both hands, arms extended in front of you.

2. **Execution:** Slowly rotate your torso to one side, keeping your arms extended and your back straight.
3. **Hold:** Pause for a second at the end of the movement.
4. **Return:** Rotate back to the starting position in a controlled manner.
5. **Repetitions:** Perform 10-15 repetitions on each side. For added challenge, use a band with higher resistance or increase the number of repetitions.

Standing Side Crunch

Standing side crunches target the obliques and improve lateral stability.

1. **Starting Position:** Stand with your feet hip-width apart, placing a loop band around your thighs just above your knees. Place your hands behind your head.
2. **Execution:** Lift one knee toward your elbow on the same side, crunching your torso sideways.
3. **Hold:** Pause for a second at the top of the movement.
4. **Return:** Lower your leg back to the starting position.
5. **Repetitions:** Perform 10-15 repetitions on each side. Use a band with higher resistance for added difficulty.

Seated Knee Tucks

Seated knee tucks strengthen the lower abs and improve overall core stability.

1. **Starting Position:** Sit on a sturdy chair with your back straight

and feet flat on the floor. Place a loop band around your thighs just above your knees.

2. **Execution:** Lift both knees toward your chest, contracting your abs.
3. **Hold:** Pause for a second at the top of the movement.
4. **Return:** Lower your legs back to the starting position.
5. **Repetitions:** Perform 10-15 repetitions. For added challenge, hold the top position for a longer period.

Plank with Resistance Bands

Planks are excellent for overall core strength and stability. Adding a resistance band increases the intensity of the exercise.

1. **Starting Position:** Get into a plank position with your forearms on the ground and your body in a straight line. Place a loop band around your wrists.
2. **Execution:** Hold the plank position, ensuring your back is straight and your core is engaged.
3. **Hold:** Maintain the position for 15-30 seconds, gradually increasing the duration as you build strength.
4. **Return:** Lower your body to the ground in a controlled manner.
5. **Repetitions:** Perform 3-5 repetitions. For added challenge, increase the resistance of the band or the duration of the hold.

Benefits for Stability and Balance

Strengthening your core has numerous benefits, especially for seniors. A strong core improves balance by stabilizing your body, which reduces the risk of falls and enhances your ability to perform daily activities safely. It also promotes better posture by strengthening the muscles that support your spine, thus reducing the risk of back pain. Additionally, core exercises enhance mobility by enabling more efficient and controlled movement, improving your overall range of motion. Furthermore, a strong core provides a solid foundation for all other movements, increasing your overall strength and physical performance. By focusing on core strengthening, you can significantly enhance your stability, balance, and overall functionality.

7

Flexibility and Stretching

The Importance of Flexibility and Stretching

Maintaining flexibility is essential for overall mobility and preventing injuries. Stretching exercises can improve your range of motion, reduce muscle tension, and enhance your ability to perform daily activities with ease. This chapter will guide you through various flexibility and stretching exercises designed for seniors, providing detailed instructions and step-by-step guidance.

Stretching Routines for Seniors

Neck Stretch

The neck stretch helps to release tension and improve flexibility in your neck and shoulders.

1. **Starting Position:** Sit or stand with your back straight and feet shoulder-width apart.

2. **Execution:** Slowly tilt your head to one side, bringing your ear towards your shoulder. Use your hand to gently press down for a deeper stretch.
3. **Hold:** Pause for 15-20 seconds, feeling the stretch along the side of your neck.
4. **Return:** Slowly return your head to the starting position.
5. **Repetitions:** Perform 2-3 repetitions on each side.

Shoulder Stretch

This stretch improves flexibility in your shoulders and upper back.

1. **Starting Position:** Sit or stand with your back straight and feet shoulder-width apart.
2. **Execution:** Extend one arm across your body at shoulder height. Use your opposite hand to press your arm closer to your chest.
3. **Hold:** Pause for 15-20 seconds, feeling the stretch in your shoulder.
4. **Return:** Slowly return your arm to the starting position.
5. **Repetitions:** Perform 2-3 repetitions on each side.

Seated Hamstring Stretch

The seated hamstring stretch targets the muscles in the back of your thighs, improving flexibility and reducing tightness.

1. **Starting Position:** Sit on the edge of a sturdy chair with one leg extended straight out in front of you, heel on the floor.
2. **Execution:** Lean forward from your hips, reaching towards your toes. Keep your back straight and avoid rounding your spine.
3. **Hold:** Pause for 15-20 seconds, feeling the stretch in your hamstring.

4. **Return:** Slowly sit back up to the starting position.
5. **Repetitions:** Perform 2-3 repetitions on each leg.

Calf Stretch

The calf stretch helps to improve flexibility in your lower legs, reducing muscle tightness and enhancing mobility.

1. **Starting Position:** Stand facing a wall with your hands placed against it at shoulder height.
2. **Execution:** Step one foot back, keeping it straight and your heel on the floor. Bend your front knee slightly and lean forward.
3. **Hold:** Pause for 15-20 seconds, feeling the stretch in your calf.
4. **Return:** Step forward to return to the starting position.
5. **Repetitions:** Perform 2-3 repetitions on each leg.

Seated Spinal Twist

The seated spinal twist improves flexibility in your spine and helps to relieve lower back tension.

1. **Starting Position:** Sit on a sturdy chair with your back straight and feet flat on the floor.
2. **Execution:** Place one hand on the back of the chair and twist your torso to that side, keeping your back straight.
3. **Hold:** Pause for 15-20 seconds, feeling the stretch along your spine.
4. **Return:** Slowly return to the starting position.
5. **Repetitions:** Perform 2-3 repetitions on each side.

Enhancing Flexibility with Bands

Using resistance bands to enhance flexibility can provide a gentle yet effective way to improve your range of motion and reduce muscle tension. Here are some easy-to-understand, step-by-step exercises using resistance bands to help seniors increase their flexibility safely and effectively.

Hamstring Stretch with Band

This stretch targets the muscles in the back of your thighs, improving flexibility and reducing tightness.

1. **Starting Position:** Lie on your back with one leg extended straight on the floor and the other leg lifted. Loop the resistance band around the arch of your lifted foot.
2. **Execution:** Hold the ends of the band in both hands and gently pull your leg towards you, keeping it straight.
3. **Hold:** Pause for 15-20 seconds, feeling the stretch in your hamstring.
4. **Return:** Slowly lower your leg back to the starting position.
5. **Repetitions:** Perform 2-3 repetitions on each leg.

Quadriceps Stretch with Band

This stretch targets the muscles in the front of your thighs, helping to improve flexibility and reduce muscle tension.

1. **Starting Position:** Lie on your side with your legs stacked. Loop the resistance band around the arch of your top foot and hold the ends with your hand.

2. **Execution:** Gently pull your foot towards your buttocks, bending your knee.
3. **Hold:** Pause for 15-20 seconds, feeling the stretch in your quadriceps.
4. **Return:** Slowly release your foot back to the starting position.
5. **Repetitions:** Perform 2-3 repetitions on each leg.

Chest Opener with Band

This stretch helps to open up the chest and improve flexibility in the shoulders and upper back.

1. **Starting Position:** Stand with your feet shoulder-width apart, holding the resistance band with both hands behind your back.
2. **Execution:** Gently pull the band apart, lifting your arms slightly to open your chest.
3. **Hold:** Pause for 15-20 seconds, feeling the stretch in your chest and shoulders.
4. **Return:** Slowly bring your arms back to the starting position.
5. **Repetitions:** Perform 2-3 repetitions.

Seated Forward Bend with Band

This stretch targets the lower back and hamstrings, helping to improve flexibility and reduce tension.

1. **Starting Position:** Sit on the floor with your legs extended straight in front of you. Loop the resistance band around the arches of both feet.
2. **Execution:** Hold the ends of the band in both hands and gently pull your upper body forward, reaching towards your toes.

3. **Hold:** Pause for 15-20 seconds, feeling the stretch in your lower back and hamstrings.
4. **Return:** Slowly sit back up to the starting position.
5. **Repetitions:** Perform 2-3 repetitions.

8

Cool Down and Recovery

The Importance of Cooling Down

Cooling down after a workout is just as important as warming up. It helps your body transition back to a resting state, reducing muscle stiffness and soreness, and preventing injury. Cooling down gradually lowers your heart rate and stretches your muscles, promoting flexibility and recovery. This chapter will guide you through the importance of cooling down and provide gentle exercises and stretches to help you recover after your workouts.

Gentle Exercises and Stretches

Gentle Marching in Place

This exercise helps to gradually lower your heart rate and relax your muscles.

1. **Starting Position:** Stand with your feet shoulder-width apart.

2. **Execution:** Slowly lift your knees in a marching motion, keeping the movement gentle and controlled.
3. **Duration:** Continue for 1-2 minutes, gradually reducing the intensity.

Shoulder Rolls

Shoulder rolls release tension in your shoulders and upper back, promoting relaxation.

1. **Starting Position:** Stand or sit with your back straight and feet shoulder-width apart.
2. **Execution:** Lift your shoulders towards your ears, then roll them back and down in a circular motion.
3. **Repetitions:** Perform 10-15 rolls, then reverse the direction for another 10-15 rolls.

Chest Stretch

This stretch helps to open up the chest and improve flexibility in the shoulders and upper back.

1. **Starting Position:** Stand with your feet shoulder-width apart, holding your arms behind your back.
2. **Execution:** Gently pull your arms back and lift your chest upwards, feeling the stretch in your chest and shoulders.
3. **Hold:** Pause for 15-20 seconds.
4. **Return:** Slowly release your arms back to the starting position.

Seated Hamstring Stretch

The seated hamstring stretch targets the muscles in the back of your thighs, helping to reduce tightness and improve flexibility.

1. **Starting Position:** Sit on the edge of a sturdy chair with one leg extended straight out in front of you, heel on the floor.
2. **Execution:** Lean forward from your hips, reaching towards your toes while keeping your back straight.
3. **Hold:** Pause for 15-20 seconds, feeling the stretch in your hamstring.
4. **Return:** Slowly sit back up to the starting position.
5. **Repetitions:** Perform 2-3 repetitions on each leg.

Calf Stretch

The calf stretch helps to reduce muscle tightness in your lower legs, enhancing mobility and preventing soreness.

1. **Starting Position:** Stand facing a wall with your hands placed against it at shoulder height.
2. **Execution:** Step one foot back, keeping it straight and your heel on the floor. Bend your front knee slightly and lean forward.
3. **Hold:** Pause for 15-20 seconds, feeling the stretch in your calf.
4. **Return:** Step forward to return to the starting position.
5. **Repetitions:** Perform 2-3 repetitions on each leg.

Cat-Cow Stretch

This stretch improves flexibility in your spine and helps to relieve tension in your back.

1. **Starting Position:** Get on your hands and knees in a tabletop position.
2. **Execution (Cat):** Arch your back towards the ceiling, tucking your chin to your chest.
3. **Hold:** Pause for a few seconds.
4. **Execution (Cow):** Lower your back towards the floor, lifting your head and tailbone towards the ceiling.
5. **Hold:** Pause for a few seconds.
6. **Repetitions:** Perform 10-15 repetitions, alternating between cat and cow.

9

Maintaining Motivation

Staying Motivated on Your Fitness Journey

Staying motivated is key to maintaining a consistent exercise routine. It's common to experience ups and downs in motivation, but with the right strategies, you can stay on track and achieve your fitness goals. This chapter will provide tips for staying consistent and setting achievable fitness goals to help you maintain your motivation.

Tips for Staying Consistent

Find an Exercise Buddy

Working out with a friend can make exercise more enjoyable and hold you accountable. You're more likely to stick with your routine if you know someone else is counting on you.

Schedule Your Workouts

Treat your exercise sessions like important appointments. Set a specific time for your workouts and add them to your calendar. Consistency in scheduling helps build a habit.

Keep It Fun

Choose activities you enjoy to make exercise something you look forward to. Whether it's dancing, gardening, or walking in the park, finding joy in movement will help keep you motivated.

Track Your Progress

Keep a fitness journal or use an app to log your workouts and track your progress. Seeing your improvements over time can be incredibly motivating and encourage you to keep going.

Reward Yourself

Set up a reward system for reaching small milestones. Treat yourself to something you enjoy, like a new book, a relaxing bath, or a special outing. Rewards can provide extra motivation to stay consistent.

Setting Achievable Fitness Goals

Start Small

Begin with small, manageable goals that are realistic for your current fitness level. This could be something as simple as taking a 10-minute walk each day. Achieving small goals builds confidence and sets the foundation for bigger accomplishments.

Be Specific

Set specific, clear goals rather than vague ones. For example, instead of saying, "I want to get fit," say, "I want to walk 30 minutes a day, five times a week." Specific goals are easier to track and measure.

Set Short-Term and Long-Term Goals

Having both short-term and long-term goals can provide a clear roadmap for your fitness journey. Short-term goals offer immediate targets to work towards, while long-term goals give you something to strive for over time.

Make Your Goals Measurable

Ensure your goals are measurable so you can track your progress. Use metrics like time, distance, or frequency to quantify your goals. For instance, aim to increase your walking distance by a certain amount each week.

Adjust Goals as Needed

Be flexible and adjust your goals as needed. If you find a goal too challenging or too easy, modify it to better suit your current abilities and circumstances. The key is to keep progressing without becoming overwhelmed.

Celebrate Your Successes

Take time to celebrate your achievements, no matter how small. Recognizing your successes reinforces your efforts and motivates you to continue working towards your goals.

Maintaining motivation is crucial for a consistent exercise routine. By finding an exercise buddy, scheduling your workouts, keeping it fun, tracking your progress, rewarding yourself, and joining a class, you can stay consistent. Setting achievable fitness goals, starting small, being specific, and celebrating your successes will keep you motivated on your fitness journey. In the next chapter, we will summarise the key points covered in this book and provide final tips for your continued success.

10

Conclusion

Wrapping Up Your Fitness Journey

Congratulations on taking the initiative to improve your strength and flexibility with resistance band workouts. This book has provided you with the tools and knowledge to embark on a fitness journey tailored to your needs. Let's recap the key points and look at how you can continue to build on your progress.

Key Takeaways

We began by discussing the importance of choosing the right resistance bands and basic equipment, ensuring you have a safe and effective start. Warm-up routines set the stage for your workouts, reducing the risk of injury and preparing your body for physical activity.

Upper body workouts focused on strengthening your shoulders, arms, and chest, providing detailed, step-by-step exercises. Lower body workouts target your legs, hips, and glute, enhancing your mobility and stability.

Core strengthening exercises were highlighted for their role in improving balance and overall stability, crucial for daily activities. Flexibility and stretching routines were emphasized to maintain and enhance your range of motion, reduce muscle tension, and prevent injuries.

Full-body workouts combine various exercises to offer a comprehensive fitness routine. Cool down and recovery exercises were detailed to ensure proper muscle relaxation and recovery post-workout.

Finally, we discussed maintaining motivation with practical tips and the importance of setting achievable fitness goals. Staying motivated and consistent is key to long-term success in your fitness journey.

Moving Forward

As you continue your fitness journey, remember to listen to your body and progress at your own pace. Consistency is more important than intensity. Regular, moderate exercise will yield significant benefits over time.

Celebrate your successes, no matter how small. Each step forward is a step towards better health and improved quality of life. Don't hesitate to revisit sections of this book as needed to refresh your memory and refine your techniques.

Final Thoughts

Your dedication to improving your strength and flexibility is commendable. By incorporating these resistance band exercises into your routine, you are investing in your health and well-being. Keep moving, stay motivated, and enjoy the journey to a stronger, more flexible you. Remember, it's never too late to start, and every effort you make brings you closer to your fitness goals. Thank you for allowing this book to be a part of your journey. Stay active and stay healthy!

Resource

Foster, M., & Lanquist, L. (2024b, May 10). Tested & Trainer-Approved: The 10 Best Resistance Bands, Plus 7 More We Like. *Verywell Fit.* https://www.verywellfit.com/best-resistance-bands-4157960

The most effective Warm-Up. (2014, March 27). https://www.acefitness.org/resources/everyone/blog/3789/the-most-effective-warm-up/

Ayuda, T., & CPT, C. S. (2021, July 31). This upper body circuit workout uses just a resistance band to smoke your shoulders, back, and arms. *SELF.* https://www.self.com/gallery/upper-body-circuit-workout-resistance-bands

Robinson, L., Segal, J., PhD, & Smith, M., MA. (2024, February 5). How to start exercising and stick to it - HelpGuide.org. *HelpGuide.org.* https://www.helpguide.org/articles/healthy-living/how-to-start-exercising-and-stick-to-it.htm